Annil Dhingra
Panna Mangat
Gaurav Bhardwaj

Light Cure Units

AF138177

Annil Dhingra
Panna Mangat
Gaurav Bhardwaj

Light Cure Units

LAP LAMBERT Academic Publishing

Impressum / Imprint

Bibliografische Information der Deutschen Nationalbibliothek: Die Deutsche Nationalbibliothek verzeichnet diese Publikation in der Deutschen Nationalbibliografie; detaillierte bibliografische Daten sind im Internet über http://dnb.d-nb.de abrufbar.
Alle in diesem Buch genannten Marken und Produktnamen unterliegen warenzeichen-, marken- oder patentrechtlichem Schutz bzw. sind Warenzeichen oder eingetragene Warenzeichen der jeweiligen Inhaber. Die Wiedergabe von Marken, Produktnamen, Gebrauchsnamen, Handelsnamen, Warenbezeichnungen u.s.w. in diesem Werk berechtigt auch ohne besondere Kennzeichnung nicht zu der Annahme, dass solche Namen im Sinne der Warenzeichen- und Markenschutzgesetzgebung als frei zu betrachten wären und daher von jedermann benutzt werden dürften.

Bibliographic information published by the Deutsche Nationalbibliothek: The Deutsche Nationalbibliothek lists this publication in the Deutsche Nationalbibliografie; detailed bibliographic data are available in the Internet at http://dnb.d-nb.de.
Any brand names and product names mentioned in this book are subject to trademark, brand or patent protection and are trademarks or registered trademarks of their respective holders. The use of brand names, product names, common names, trade names, product descriptions etc. even without a particular marking in this work is in no way to be construed to mean that such names may be regarded as unrestricted in respect of trademark and brand protection legislation and could thus be used by anyone.

Coverbild / Cover image: www.ingimage.com

Verlag / Publisher:
LAP LAMBERT Academic Publishing
ist ein Imprint der / is a trademark of
OmniScriptum GmbH & Co. KG
Heinrich-Böcking-Str. 6-8, 66121 Saarbrücken, Deutschland / Germany
Email: info@lap-publishing.com

Herstellung: siehe letzte Seite /
Printed at: see last page
ISBN: 978-3-8484-9063-9

Copyright © 2015 OmniScriptum GmbH & Co. KG
Alle Rechte vorbehalten. / All rights reserved. Saarbrücken 2015

"LIGHT CURE UNITS"

Authors

Dr Panna Mangat

Reader

Department of Conservative Dentistry & Endodontics

D.J. College of Dental Sciences & Research

Modinagar, U.P (India)

Dr Annil Dhingra

B.D.S., M.D.S., F.A.G.E., F.I.C.D.

Professor & Head

Department of Conservative Dentistry & Endodontics

D.J College Of Dental Sciences & Research

Modinagar, U.P (India)

Dr. Gaurav Bhardwaj

Post Graduate Student

Department of Conservative Dentisrty & Endodontics

D.J College Of Dental Sciences & Research

Modinagar, U.P (India)

Corresponding Address

E-mail: gauravendo1987@gmail.com

Background

Since the inception of dentistry, continuous attempts have been made to devise a material and technique that fulfills aesthetic requirements, besides having the expected physical, mechanical, and biological properties to behave favorably in the oral environment. Clinical efficiency of a light-curing unit is crucial for obtaining the optimal polymerization and a successful outcome[1]. With the research in the field of restorative materials, a need for an appropriate curing unit has always been felt.

Usually, visible light–cured (VLC) composite materials use α-1,2-diketone (benzyl or camphorquinone) as a free radical initiator and an amine-reducing agent (dimethylaminoethyl methacrylate). Intense visible light in the 400–500 nm range is used to transform the diketone to its excited state, thus producing free radicals. As the light passes through the composite, it is absorbed and scattered leaving layers more remote from the surface with considerable residual unsaturation[2].

Three major evolutions in dental composite curing lights have occurred since 1991. At that time, the majority of practitioners used quartz–tungsten–halogen units with power densities in the 400–600 mW/cm^2 range.

Many attempts have been made to improve their physical and mechanical properties, such as hardness and curing time, by improvising the polymerization process.

According to Safarcherati and Alaghehmand[3], surface hardness can be defined as resistance to surface indentation, which is an indirect method for measuring degree of polymerization. The comparison of hardness between the deep parts and the surface provides valuable information. Because polymerization of light-curing resins depends on source and properties of light source, improvement in light-curing units can enhance the properties of final restoration[4]. According to some studies, when a light source is placed at a distance of more than 6 mm, the polymerization of composites gets affected, whereas at a distance of 12 mm, no appropriate curing could be achieved. Thus, curing depths and curing time also contribute to the polymerization of composite resins.

Curing Lamps/Curing Units

Four types of light sources can be used in the polymerization of light-curable dental materials:

1. Quartz–tungsten–halogen curing lights
2. Light-emitting diode curing lights
3. Plasma arc curing lights
4. Laser curing lights

Quartz–tungsten–halogen curing lights

For many years, quartz–tungsten–halogen lamps have been the standard curing units, irrespective of a remarkably low efficiency compared to heat-generation unit. With these, of the total energy, 5% is visible light, 12% is heat, and 80% is light emitted in the infrared spectrum. Normally, a halogen bulb combined with a filter is the source of blue light, which lies in the 410–500 nm region of the visible spectrum. Light in this range of wavelengths is most effectively absorbed by camphorquinone photoinitiator present in the resin component of light-activated dental composites. This light excites camphorquinone, which in combination with an amine produces free radicals. This results in polymerization of resin monomers at the molecular scale. It usually takes 20–60 s for polymerization to take place macroscopically.

Light-emitting diode curing lights

Mills introduced light-emitting diode technology in 1995 to polymerize light-activated dental materials[5]. The spectral emittance of gallium nitride–based blue light–emitting diodes covers the absorption spectrum of camphorquinone so that no filters are required in light-emitting diode light-curing units[6]. Recent reports have shown that blue light–emitting diode lamps offer the highest photopolymerization efficiency[7]. Light-emitting diodes use junctions of doped semiconductors for generating light, have a lifetime of more than 10,000 h, undergo little degradation of output over time, are resistant to shock and vibration, and consume little power on operation. The newer gallium nitride–based light-emitting diodes produce a narrow spectrum of light (400–500 nm) that falls closely within the absorption range of camphorquinone, which initiates the polymerization of resin monomers[8].

Plasma arc curing lights

Plasma arc curing lamps emit light at higher intensities and were primarily designed to save irradiation time as an economic factor. They typically produce power density of more than 2000 mW/cm^2 and have shown to polymerize composite in the least amount of time. Owing to the described high-energy output of plasma arc systems, the manufacturers of these lamps claim that 3-s irradiation from plasma arc curing lamps would achieve material properties similar to that achieved through 40 s curing with quartz–tungsten–halogen lamps[9].

Laser curing lights

Dental lasers were introduced and recognized as a tool for better patient care in the early 1990s. The argon laser (with wavelength between 450 and 500 nm) can be used effectively to polymerize composite resins because it enhances the physical properties of the restorative material compared with conventional VLC. Lasers produce little heat, because of limited infrared output[9]

According to Strassler[4], the first light-curing resin composites were introduced in the early 1960s, eventually leading to the development of the first curing light (Fig. 1).

Nuva Light (Dentsply/Caulk) was the first dental curing light developed in the 1970s, which used ultraviolet (UV) light to cure the material. These lights were discontinued because of UV light use and less effectiveness as a result of shorter wavelengths that limited the depth of cure.

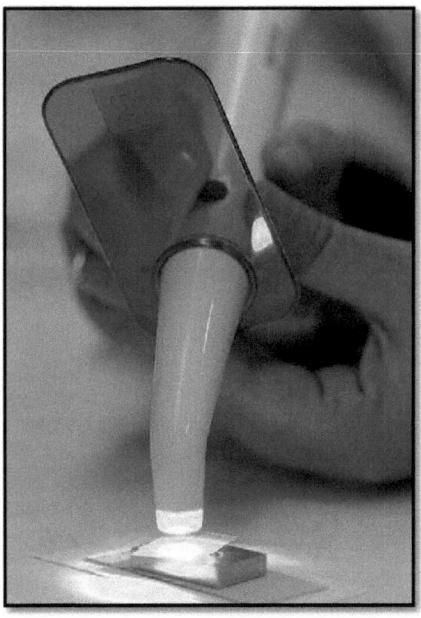

Fig. 1. Curing of composite by light-curing unit

According to Rueggeberg[10], advances in the area of visible light curing took place in the early 1980s. Only a few years after the introduction of UV radiation for curing dental restoratives, visible radiation was introduced: February 24, 1976. On that day, Dr Mohammed Bassoiuny of the Turner

School of Dentistry, Manchester, placed the first visible light–cured composite restoration on Dr John Yearn, the then head of department. This advancement led to a curing device that now uses blue light. Next the quartz–halogen bulb was developed, which had longer wavelengths of the visible light spectrum and allowed for greater penetrating curing light and light energy. The halogen curing light replaced the UV curing light.

Initially, the quartz–tungsten–halogen light source was developed by engineers at General Electric for use in aircraft lights, where small but very bright and durable sources were needed. However, into the late 1990s, it became the mainstay of dental light curing. During that time advances included a wide range of adaptations for convenience and efficacy.

The 1990s presented great improvements in light-curing devices, both previous and developing new devices. As there were advancements with dental restorative materials, the technology to cure these materials also improved. The prime focus was to improve the intensity to be able to cure faster and deeper.

The plasma arc curing light was introduced in 1998. It uses a high-intensity fluorescent bulb containing plasma to cure the resin-based composite. Although it claimed to be able to cure material in 3 s, on average it took between 3 and 5 s. Because dental auxiliaries were prohibited from using the argon laser in the United States, technology (i.e., the plasma arc curing light) was imported from Europe (French patent 2,305,092, 1976), where it had already met with a great amount of success. Developed in the mid-1960s, this was not initially developed for dental purposes, but was used to provide broad-banded radiation for visualization of operating fields (e.g., endoscopy and colonoscopy) as well as for minimally invasive medical procedures.

This light was highly popular but the negatives outweighed the positives. The initial price was three times higher than that of the halogen and light-emitting diode lights. Also, its maintenance was expensive. The latest advancement in technology comes with the light-emitting diode curing light, which has been available for the past 14 years but was put into use at the turn of the twenty-first century. Advances in this technology are still taking place.

Nature has provided us with diverse forms of composites, such as wood, which are known as *natural composite materials*. Wood consists of one species of polymer-cellulose fibers with good strength and stiffness in a resinous matrix of another polymer, the polysaccharide lignin. Since ancient times, humans have been aware of the concept of combining materials advantageously. The extremely simple procedures of wattle and daub (mud and straw) and "pide" (heather incorporated in hard-rammed earth), which are being used even today, actually predate the use of reinforced concrete by the Romans that foreshadowed the pre- and post-tensioned reinforced concretes of the recent times.

Our bones are also composites. Bone comprises hard but brittle material called hydroxyapatite (calcium phosphate) and soft and flexible material called collagen (a protein). The first modern composite material was fiberglass, which is still widely used for boat hulls, sports equipment, building panels, and many vehicle bodies. The matrix is a plastic and the reinforcement is glass that has been made into fine threads and often woven into a sort of cloth. The glass is very strong but brittle, so it will break easily if bent sharply. Here, the plastic matrix holds the glass fibers together and also protects them from damage.

Why composites?

The biggest advantage of composites is that they are light but still strong. We can easily make a new material meeting our requirements by selecting appropriate combination of matrix and filler.

Various composite materials are available nowadays for direct restorative techniques, most well known being hybrid composites. This technology, which is based on methacrylates and different types of filler coupled with silanes, is being continuously improved.

Despite these advancements, disadvantages of composites such as polymerization shrinkage, bacterial adhesion, and side effects due to monomer release still remain. The material development aims to eliminate or at least reduce these negative factors by adapting the individual components of the material. With ormocers, the methacrylate has been partially replaced by an inorganic network. According to recent studies, the biocompatibility could not be improved in all cases.

An example of composite technology is the development of compomer, combining the positive properties of glass ionomers. This has only partially succeeded, as the release of fluoride is low. In an *in situ* study, caries protective effect could be shown at least in the first few days after filling placement with concurrent extraoral demineralization. A new approach to reduce polymerization shrinkage was substituting the chain monomers in the composite matrix with ring-shaped molecules.

In the past decade, several alternative preparations to the traditional GV Black cavity preparations have been suggested, which are much smaller in size than the conventional cavity preparations and are thus termed "microconservatives"[10]. The cavity design modification is essential because the conventional cavity requires extension, which has been increasingly questioned and seems unnecessary as fissure sealants are now available. Extension for retention has also become unnecessary because of the availability of adhesive restoration materials. Because materials such as composite resins are available, which can provide reinforcement, extension to remove weakened tooth structure is now unnecessary.

Hunt[11] introduced an "internal" preparation technique that involved access to the carious lesion form, an occlusal approach just inside the marginal ridge; removal of the carious dentine via this occlusal cavity; and finally, handling the proximal enamel lesion. The three methods of handling the enamel lesion are as follows: (1) punching or drilling out the weakened or porous enamel; (2) leaving intact the enamel porosity to avoid trauma to the enamel wall and to retain a shell of porous enamel, permitting remineralization; and (3) cutting a minibox to remove the porous enamel, and at the same time removing the overlying enamel up to and including a portion of the enamel ridge.

Three main components of composites are the following: (1) resin matrix, a plastic resin material that forms a continuous phase and binds the filler particles; (2) filler, reinforcing particles or fibers that are dispersed in the matrix; and (3) coupling agent, a bonding agent that promotes adhesion between filler and resin matrix.

Restoration techniques

To reduce the effect of polymerization shrinkage and contraction stresses, specific filling techniques have been introduced for composite resin restorations. Studies have shown that light-cured composite resins shrink in the direction of the polymerization light source[3]. Contraction toward the light source causes the resin to shrink from margins of the preparation.

Park et al.[12] used the following three restoration techniques and studied the three groups for shrinkage:

1. *Bulk filling technique (Group 1)*: Composite was placed in one increment and light cured from the upper surface for 40 s, the mesial side for 20 s, and the distal side for 20 s (total 80 s).

2. *Horizontal incremental technique (Group 2)*: Composite was placed in three horizontal consecutive layers. Each increment was light cured for 20 s and additionally for 20 s from the upper surface to make curing time identical (total 80 s).

3. *Oblique incremental technique (Group 3)*: Composite was placed in three oblique increments with each increment being light cured for 20 s followed by an additional 20-s curing from the upper surface.

Various resin composite "sandwich" restorations have been proposed. In a sandwich restoration, the resin composite is replaced by another material with lower elastic modulus in the dentin part of the cavity. A sandwich restoration can either be closed or open. In both the closed- and the open-sandwich restorations, the first horizontal layer can be conventional glass ionomer cement, resin-modified glass ionomer cement, polyacid-modified resin composite, or flowable resin composite. In the closed-sandwich restoration, the first layer is completely covered by the resin composite, whereas in the open-sandwich restoration the first layer reaches the outer cervical margins.

Lutz *et al.*[13] introduced the "three-sited light-curing technique" that was used in conjunction with light-reflecting wedges. In this technique, the polymerization was intended to be guided toward the cervical cavity margins through light-conducting wedges and with a direct curing through the cusps, which was considered to result in better marginal adaptation. This technique, though complex, was found to minimize the adverse effects of composite resin polymerization shrinkage. Therefore, this was recommended for use in Class II restorations.

Another study by Ciucchi *et al.*[14] compared the proximal adaptation and the marginal seal of various posterior composite resin restorations using different filling techniques. The following are the three filling techniques used by them: the three-sited light-curing technique, the multilayer technique, and the indirect composite inlay technique. The results did not show statistically significant differences in adaptation or marginal seal among the three composites. A new group of materials, the siloranes, has been developed. Since siloranes are hydrophobic they need to be bonded to the dental hard tissue using a special adhesive system. Long-term clinical studies are still needed to prove the superiority of siloranes over modern hybrid composites.

Silorane

The name Silorane is derived from its chemical building blocks siloxanes and oxiranes. This material class aims to have lower shrinkage, longer resistance to fading, and less marginal discoloration. The silorane monomer ring differs obviously from the chain-monomers of hybrid composites. The hydrophobic properties of the material (reduction in exogenous discoloration and water absorption) are due to siloxanes. The physical properties and the low shrinkage of the material are due to the oxirane rings. Cationic reactions polymerize siloranes in contrast to methacrylates, which cross-link via radicals. The photoinitiator system is based on three components: light-absorbing camphor chinon, an electron donor (e.g., amine), and an iodonium salt. When the camphor chinon is excited, it reacts with the electron donor, thus reducing the iodonium salt to an acidic cation. This leads the opening of the oxirane ring. To some extent, the polymerization shrinkage is compensated by the ring opening of the oxirane during the polymerization process. The fillers in Filtek Silorane-R, the only silorane material on the market at the moment, are composed of quartz particles (0.1–2.0 μm) and radiopaque yttrium fluoride.

Polymerization Reaction

In general, light-cured dental composites are supplied in a single-paste, lightproof syringe. This paste has a free radical initiating system, which comprises a photosensitizer and an amine initiator. When unexposed to light, the two components remain unreactive. However, on exposure to light in the blue region, the photosensitizer gets excited, leading to the formation of free radicals. Thus, an addition polymerization reaction is initiated.

Camphorquinone (CQ) is the most widely used photosensitizer that absorbs blue light between 400 and 500 nm. An amine initiator (such as dimethylaminoethyl methacrylate) is used in low quantities (0.15 wt.%). CQ is required in as low as 0.2 wt.%. The process of polymerization has been shown in a flowchart.

Polymerization reaction

Light activates the photoinitiator system in the light-curing unit.

Activated photoinitiator system then starts the polymerization reaction. In a first approximation, each activated photoinitiator stays active for a certain period.

Activated photoinitiator integrates a number of monomers into polymer network.

The photoinitiator molecule gets activated by absorbing a photon.

The absorbed energy is then used to change the molecular structure that forms a radical.

Absorption of light by the molecule leads to the activation of photoinitiator. The number of activated photoinitiator molecules depends on the amount of photoinitiator present in the sample. This amount of photoinitiator is defined by the manufacturer, whereas the number and energy of photons is decided by the design of the light-curing unit. Maximum absorption occurs at 470 nm for CQ.

The equation for correlation between number of photons and light intensity is as follows:

$$\text{Dose} = \text{Intensity} \times \text{Time}$$

The activated photoinitiator is nothing but a radical, which attaches and activates the monomer. Similarly, monomers attach to each other resulting in a growing polymer chain. Theoretically, this process can go on and on, however practically, certain chemicals and radicals are present that stop the chain reaction after some time. Usually, a radical in a reaction stays active for about 0.1–1.0 s.

During this reaction, around 50 monomers are integrated into the polymer network. Although the effect of oxygen and stabilizers on the polymerization process is independent of light intensity, the amount of activated photoinitiator depends on intensity. An activated photoinitiator not only can start a reaction but also can stop a chain reaction with an activated end of polymer chain. A higher light dose is needed to get the same degree of polymerization.

Ideal Requirements for Light-Curing Units

The ideal requirements for a light-curing unit are broad emission spectrum, sufficient light intensity, minimal decline of energy with distance, multiple curing modes, sufficient duration for multiple curing cycles, durability, large curing footprint, and ease of repair[14].

Types of Light-Curing Unit

Three types of light-curing unit are as follows:

1. Countertop unit

2. Gun-type unit

3. Fiber-optic handpiece curing attachment

Countertop unit

These types of light-curing units contain all the functional parts in a single box. A cord (fiber-optic or fluid-filled) carries the light from the box to the patient. Some of these units have a control switch at the end of the cord, so the operator does not have to leave the operating field to activate the light source.

Advantages

- The fan and working parts of the unit are out of the operating field.
- They are generally less expensive than other designs.

Disadvantages

- Many units lack a switch at the cord end.
- Many models do not have wide diameter curing tips.
- Many units with fiber-optic cords need periodic replacement because of fiber-optic bundle break down[9].

Gun-type unit

These types of units have a gun handle; the light passes through a small fiber-optic cord or glass rod that forms the barrel of the gun; are generally attached to an additional tabletop or wall-mounted unit that contains the necessary transformers to operate the light; and are activated at the operator site.

Advantages

- They typically have large diameters of cure with good intensity.
- They are generally small and can be easily made portable.

Disadvantages

- They have no fiber-optic cords to be replaced because the gun barrels are usually inflexible.
- The fan in the handle can be noisy and become warm with extended use.
- They are bulky, have more weight (more bulky than fiber-optic cord ends), and are costly[9].

Fiber-optic handpiece curing attachment

These are generally adapted to existing fiber-optic handpiece light sources. Attachment units have smaller curing tips, which are similar to those in countertop units. Some of these units generate considerable heat, which is due to inefficient or missing blue light filters.

Advantages

- They are less expensive, especially if the fiber-optic handpiece is already in place.
- They are small and require no additional counterspace.

Disadvantages

- They have a smaller diameter of cure.
- They are less intense light source.
- They release excessive heat (some units).
- They need periodic replacement of fiber-optic cords.

Generations of Light-Curing Units

The following are the five generations of light-curing units:

1. First generation: Ultraviolet lights
2. Second generation: Visible light–curing units
3. Third generation: Plasma arc units
4. Fourth generation: Light-emitting diodes
5. Fifth generation: Lasers

First Generation: Ultraviolet Light-Curing Units

Application of light to polymerize resin-based materials was an existing technology that was adapted for dental use. The first photocuring units, introduced in the early 1970s, were designed to emit ultraviolet light (about 365 nm) through a quartz rod from a high-pressure mercury source (Fig. 2). In dentistry, this development was a revolutionary step allowing a "cure-on-demand" feature, which was earlier infeasible with the self-curing products. Typical exposure duration was 20 s, but 60 s provided enhanced results.

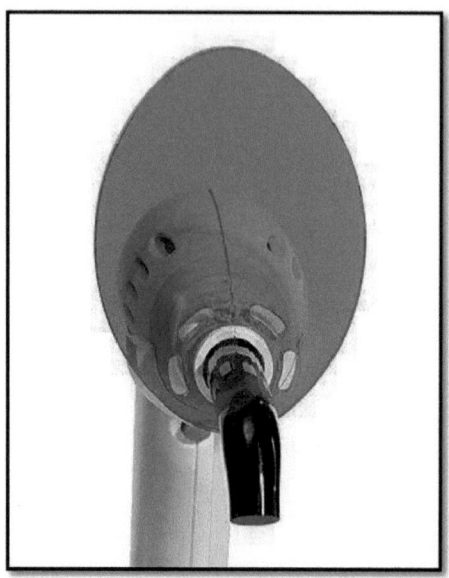

Fig. 2. Ultraviolet curing light

Filled, photocurable composites and sealant materials were available, which were used in very innovative ways to not only restore carious processes but also repair tooth fractures and provide easily performed aesthetic results. The photoinitiating system was dependent on benzoin ether–type compounds, which broke down into multiple radicals, without need of an intermediary component. The spectral distribution of light sources of the time with the absorption spectrum of the initiator helps to correlate these two parameters. Although some of the restorations placed using this early technology have proven to be remarkably successful, in general the procedure had many issues.

Disadvantages of ultraviolet light-curing units

Following are the drawbacks of this type of curing light:

1. Because of the limited ability of light to penetrate deep within the material, incremental buildups were required instead of bulk placement, and were limited in depth.

2. Short wavelength energy has harmful effects on human eyes (corneal burns and cataract formation) as well as can lead to possible changes in the oral microflora.

Second Generation: Visible Light–Curing Units (Quartz–Tungsten–Halogen Lamps)

Curing of dental composites with blue light was introduced in the 1970s[5]. Normally, blue light in the 410–500 nm region of the visible spectrum is produced using a halogen bulb combined with a filter. In this region of the spectrum, light is most effectively absorbed by the photoinitiator (camphorquinone) that is present in the resin component of light-activated dental composites, thus exciting the photoinitiator, which in combination with an amine produces free radicals. This results in molecular-scale polymerization of resin monomers.

A tungsten filament in the quartz bulb containing the halogen gas gets heated up. The light from the bulb is collected by reflecting it from a silverized mirror behind the bulb toward the path down the fiber-optic chain to the tip. It is necessary to keep the surface of the mirror clean. In the process of heating up and cooling down, vapors from mercury, bonding agent solutions, or moisture might get condensed over its surface. Alcohol or methyl ethyl ketone solvents should be used to routinely clean the surface with the help of cotton swabs to renew its effectiveness. Macroscopically, the dental composite hardens, typically after light exposure from 20 to 60 s. The blue light is delivered to the dental treatment area using various types of light guides, which may be fused rigid glass fiber bundles or molded polymer guides. Some guides use a flexible pipe containing a transparent liquid to transmit the light[4].

Halogen bulb–based light-curing units are most commonly used to cure dental composites. However, this technology has many drawbacks. Halogen bulbs have a limited effective lifetime of around 50 h[4], implicating reduction in curing efficiency over time due to aging of the components. Many quartz–tungsten–halogen lamps used in dental offices operate below the specified minimum power output. The performance of the light-curing unit, especially the light tip, may retrograde over time due to insufficient maintenance. For a dentist, the clinical implication of this is a negative effect on the physical properties of composites with an increased risk of premature failure of restorations. The lower effective limit of irradiance for halogen bulb–based light-curing units used in dental practice has been suggested to be 300 mWcm[2]. Some units available presently exceed an irradiance of 1000 mWcm[2], which can be due to insufficient maintenance by the clinicians.

Soft-Start Polymerization Technique

"Soft-start" polymerization is a method recently advocated to reduce polymerization contraction stresses in resin composite restorations[10]. During early stages of polymerization, the cross-linking network of resin composites is relatively weak allowing "flow" to easily accommodate for stresses and prevent damage to adhesive bonds. With further polymerization, contraction and flow decrease, whereas stiffness and stress increase, which may lead to adhesive failure. For a stable marginal adaptation, the bond strength must surpass the contraction stress[15]. Soft-start polymerization proposes that a slower rate of conversion will allow better flow of resin with a decrease in contraction stress.

Soft-start polymerization can be divided into three techniques:

1. *Stepped*: In this, low irradiance is emitted for around 10 s and then increases immediately to a maximum value for the duration of exposure.
2. *Ramped*: In this, the irradiance gradually increases from a low value to maximum intensity over a 10-s period, which then remains constant for the duration of exposure.
3. *Pulse delay*: This uses a short low-level burst, a delay for polishing, and finally a long exposure at full intensity.

To determine the degree of conversion (DC) of C=C bonds of the methacrylate group in resin composites, mechanical (dilatometric), calorimetric, and spectroscopy techniques can be used[16]. In principle, the latter method provides more reliable results. Spectroscopy methods provide direct measurements of the DC value, because specific vibrational bands can be used as internal standards[17]. Some molecular vibrational techniques, such as infrared spectroscopy and Raman spectroscopy, have been used to evaluate the DC produced on dental composites[18-20]. Fourier transform infrared spectroscopy (FTIR) has been used to evaluate the DC of dental composites cured by light-emitting diode and halogen lamp–based light-curing units, detecting the C=C stretching vibrations before and after curing the materials[21-23]. However, to measure the DC of bulk composite using FTIR, polymerized samples need to be powdered in a matrix.

Raman spectroscopy has also been used to study the DC of resin composites photoactivated by traditional halogen lamp sources and by argon laser beam. Although this technique is known to be nondestructive, it has a high fluorescence signal. As in the case of FTIR technique, no specific sample preparation is required in FT-Raman analysis, therefore the measurements are fairly simple and results are obtained faster. It has been used to evaluate the DC of dental composites cured by light-emitting diodes. Literature is scarce on the influence of dental composites produced by the soft-start mode of curing and by high-power light-emitting diode curing units on the DC. Also, no reports are available in the literature regarding the influence of light guide tip material on the DC of dental composites. Thus, Soares *et al.*[24] evaluated the DC in a given composite material by FT-Raman spectroscopy when cured by three light sources using soft-start and normal protocols: a conventional halogen lamp with optical fiber light guide tip, a high-power light-emitting diode unit, and a low-power light-emitting diode with two light guide tips (polymer and optical fiber).

Disadvantages of Quartz–Tungsten–Halogen Curing Light

This type of curing light however has certain drawbacks:

1. Owing to the high temperatures generated by the filament, the curing light needs to have a ventilating fan installed to "force airflow through slots in the casing". This makes the unit large.

2. The fan generates a sound that may disturb some patients, and the wattage of the bulb is such (e.g., 80 W) that these curing lights must be plugged into a power source, that is, they are not cordless.

3. Owing to high temperatures generated, it requires frequent monitoring and replacement of the actual curing light bulb. (For example, one model uses a bulb with an estimated life of 50 h, which would require annual replacement, assuming 12-min use per day, 250 days per year.)

4. The time required to cure the material completely surpasses that for the light-emitting diode curing light. This shows a reduction of curing efficiency over time as a result of component aging. Many quartz–tungsten–halogen lamps used in dental offices operate at output power much below the minimum power output specified by the manufacturers[25], leading to reduced curing depths of the materials.

Third Generation: Plasma Arc Curing Light (Fig. 3)

This unit was developed by the United States National Aeronautics and Space Association (NASA), which was used in aeronautical engineering[23]. High-intensity light is emitted by plasma arc curing lamps, and these lamps were primarily designed to save irradiation time as an economic factor. They emit light from glowing plasma, which comprised a gaseous mixture of ionized molecules such as xenon molecules and electrons[26]. They have high intensities in a narrow wavelength range of around 470 nm. Due to the high-energy output of plasma arc systems, the manufacturers of these lamps repeatedly claimed that 3 s of plasma arc curing irradiation would achieve similar material properties compared to 40 s curing with quartz–tungsten–halogen lamps. However, this claim has been fully rejected. Today, recommendations for plasma arc curing lights are based on 3 × 3 s.

Pettemerides *et al.*[27] showed that a curing time of 20 and 30 s per tooth for plasma arc curing lights had no significant difference in the bond strength when used irrespective of bonding agent. Thus, the plasma arc was found to save the clinical time for curing of dental composites.

They have a few disadvantages when compared to recent curing units available, such as they are expensive and are of relatively large sizes. It has been postulated that high-intensity plasma arc irradiation immediately starts and makes fast the progression of shrinkage strain. This could shorten the pregel period, reducing the flow capacity of the composite. This phenomenon could negatively affect the marginal adaptation of the composite restoration[28]. The lower energy dose of the plasma arc units (5.4 J/cm²) than the quartz–tungsten–halogen units (16 J/cm²) should be taken into consideration. It is well known that the lower energy dose reduces the degree of conversion, thus lowering the polymerization shrinkage.

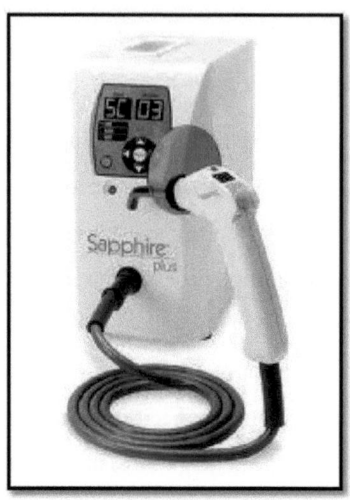

Fig. 3. DenMat Rembrandt Sapphire Light (plasma arc light)

Fourth Generation: Light-Emitting Diode Curing Units

Light-emitting diodes, such as those used as indicators in car dashboards, have lifetimes of over 10,000 h and undergo little light output degradation over this duration. Also, they require no filters to produce blue light[5]. The spectral flux of light-emitting diode is concentrated over a much narrower bandwidth than that of quartz–tungsten–halogen or plasma arc curing units. Over the past few years, several generations of light-emitting diode light-curing units (Fig. 4) have been introduced.

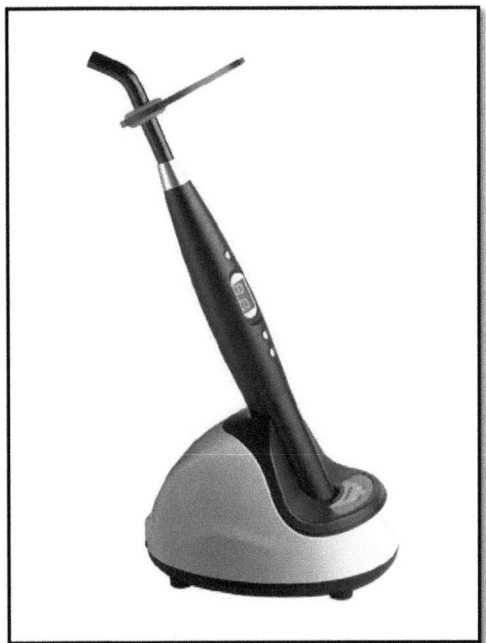

Fig. 4. Light-emitting diode curing light

Generally, the first-generation light-emitting diode light-curing units were of low intensity and were unable to cure materials completely. These "blue light" units were not able to activate the alternative photoinitiators used in bleach shades and the incisal (translucent) shades of composites and in sealants and bonding agents. The second-generation light-emitting diode light-curing units (bluephase, Elipar FreeLight 2, L.E. Demetron 1, Radii, Allegro, SmartLite iQ, the CURE) have a single, high-powered diode with multiple emission areas. These units show a large surface area of emission and high-energy output. The third-generation light-emitting diode light-curing units (UltraLume 5) have two or more diode frequencies, and they emit light in different ranges to activate CQ and alternative photoinitiators[30].

The light-emitting diodes use junctions of doped semiconductors (p–n junctions) for the generation of light. In gallium nitride (GaN) light-emitting diodes under forward biased conditions, electrons and holes recombine at the p–n junction generating blue light. A small polymer lens in front of p–n junction partially collimates the light[31]. Recently, the development of high-power light-emitting diodes is comparable to the advances we have seen in the computer technology. High-power light-emitting diodes have shown high outputs even with single diodes. However, the heat generation with these is a major concern in the clinical field.

Advances

G-Light, a curing light that uses the latest light-emitting diode technology, has been designed and manufactured by GC. The light initiator CQ is not present in many new dental materials and thus these materials cannot be cured by conventional "blue light" light-emitting diodes. Blue and violet light-emitting diodes of G-Light produce two peaks of different wavelengths simultaneously, ensuring an optimum curing of all visible light–curing units. With a high-intensity, narrow spectrum of light, it emits the maximum light energy directly to the tip of the handpiece. This rechargeable light can be used over 400 times for 10 s without any reduction in its intensity. Its constant light energy guarantees efficient and deep curing every time[54].

To determine the time taken to adequately cure a composite, energy density used has to be taken into consideration, which is the irradiance of the light multiplied by the time of application (measured in joules). The distance from the composite surface drastically affects the power generated. The collimation of the light, or the amount of light wasted when not properly focused forward, can radically affect the power at depth.

As mentioned earlier, the wavelength and the type of composite affect the light-curing efficiency. In conclusion, it takes about 17–20 J/cm^2, which equates to 20 s with a light energy of 1000 mW/cm^2 to obtain the optimum degree of polymerization of a composite. Inadequate polymerization can still occur even after the recommended curing times due to insufficient irradiance, irrespective of the technique being used and the care taken by the clinician during the process. We know that turbo tips that channel the light have poor energy at distance and in particular situations, such as very deep cavity preparations, trans-tooth curing, opaque composites, or the curing of resin cements through indirect ceramic veneers, onlays, or crowns. Corciolani et al.[33] stated that increase in the curing time is mandatory in these cases.

Fifth Generation: Lasers

Dental lasers were introduced and recognized as a tool for better patient care in the early 1990s. Argon laser (between 450 and 500 nm) has been used effectively to polymerize composite resins because it improves the physical properties of the restorative material when compared with conventional visible light–curing units. Because of limited infrared output, less heat is generated by lasers. Argon laser is useful in curing Class II composite restorations because of the decreased curing time and small fiber size, which allows for easy access of the curing light to the interproximal box area. A major drawback of arc and laser lamps is that they have a narrow light guide (or spot size). If the restoration is larger than the curing tip, the clinician had to overlap curing cycles.

Laser (light amplification by stimulated emission of radiation) light is a high-energy, coherent, unidirectional, monochromatic, and collimated beam.

Theodore H. Maiman developed the first lasers, a pulsed laser, in 1960. Since then, laser has been of keen interest in dentistry.

All lasers have an active medium that identifies them and they are usually named after the medium. Each of these medium may have different wavelengths and characteristics. The most common systems used in dentistry today are CO_2 laser, Nd:YAG laser, argon laser, holimium:YAG laser, and Er:YAG laser.

Argon laser

Conventional visible light curing units comprise white light with unwanted wavelengths filtered out, thereby producing a polychromatic spectrum of blue light. The resulting hue and brightness of the color are of wide spectrum and low intensity, respectively. In research on composite resin photopolymerization, visible light–curing units can activate CQ but optimum curing power is not achieved, and the units often are not able to meet the challenges presented by more complex resin restorations. In addition, the hue and brightness parameters of conventional visible light–curing units are not uniform over time. Bulbs, reflectors, and light tips degrade, and filter becomes baked from heat generated by the units, slowly altering the spectrum of light. Lack of predictability and consistency of restoration quality are a result of these changes. Unlike visible light–curing units, the argon laser does not use filters, instead it generates one wavelength of blue light (i.e., light is monochromatic) having a bandwidth of only 40–45 nm. In addition, for maximum efficiency, the brightness of light can be set according to the specifications by the manufacture, particular for each brand of composite resin. Some lasers can be calibrated before each cure, ensuring standard treatment for each patient.

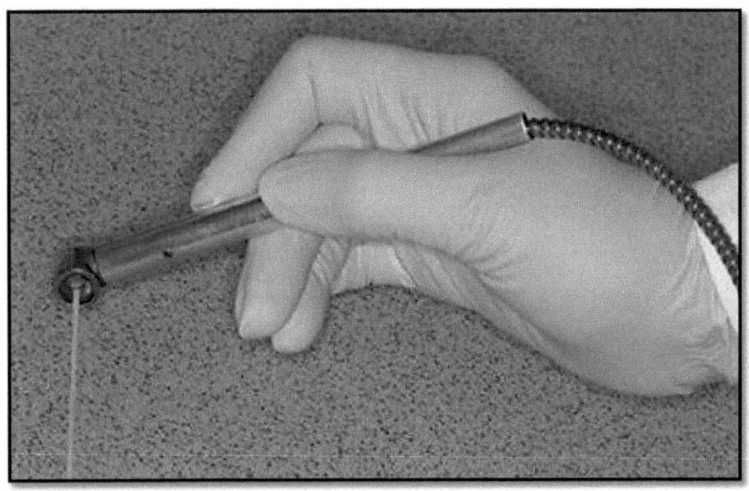

Fig. 5. Argon laser light-curing unit

Active medium for argon lasers is argon gas that is fiber-optically delivered in continuous and gated-pulse modes. This laser has two emission wavelengths that are visible to human eye: 488 nm (blue) and 514 nm (blue green). The 488-nm emission is required to activate the photoinitiator CQ. Argon laser light-curing units have much shorter curing time compared with conventional dental light units, with the advantage of having an excessive amount of photons to ensure proper cure of the material.

Laser photons travel "in phase" (i.e., are coherent), and are collimated such that they travel in the same direction. Although the output of power by the argon laser units is less than that of the conventional visible light–curing units, yet they can cure the resin more effectively because the wavelength of the light is specific to the job performed. Wide bandwidths of 120 nm of visible light–curing units result in a broad spectrum of wavelengths that overlap and are considered to be "out of phase" or incoherent[34]. Two photons of incoherent light that are 180° out of phase can cancel each other, which results in decreased curing power and less polymerization of the composite resin. A divergent beam of light produced by visible light–curing units can reduce the energy by 40% at 6 mm from the curing surface. However, lasers result in a more consistent power density over distance[35,36].

A study determined whether a GaN-based violet laser diode (VLM500) could be used as a light source for light-cured dental resins. Three experimental unfilled resins containing different photoinitiators (CQ, phenyl propanedione, or monoacylphosphine oxide) were evaluated[37], which were cured with a VLM500 laser diode, and their ultimate micro-tensile strengths (µTS) were compared to those cured with three light-emitting diode light sources (Curenos, G-Light Prima-normal mode, and G-Light Prima-PL mode). High µTS values were produced by VLM500 in all three resins, thus concluding that it can be used as a light source for light-cured dental resin materials.

Advantages

The thoroughness and depth of composite resin polymerization are greater when cured with argon laser than with visible light–curing units. Resins cured with argon laser have less unpolymerized monomer compared to those cured with visible light–curing units, enhancing its certain physical properties such as compressive strength, diametric TS, transverse flexural strength, and flexural modulus.

Wear resistance is equivalent when using either method of polymerization, but argon laser polymerization has shown the potential to improve shear bond strength in both enamel and dentin. Another study reported no significant difference in bond strengths according to distance between the resin surface and the light source. The laser-cured bond strengths were not found to decrease, whereas significant decrease in the halogen-cured bond strengths was observed at distances more than 0.5 mm. Also, laser required less time to achieve equivalent or greater polymerization of restorative material.

One manufacturer claimed that the argon laser needs only one-fourth of the exposure time: 10 s for 2-mm depth of cure compared to 40 s recommended for visible light–curing unit systems (Dentalaser Brochure 1998, Premier Laser Systems). Finally, the patient's perception and acceptance to lasers was found to be positive.

Disadvantages

Size, weight, and portability: Although size, weight, and portability of newer argon curing units have improved greatly over the older ones, at approximately 20 pounds, the unit is still fairly cumbersome and occupies considerably more space than conventional visible light–curing units[38].

Heat generation: The laser can generate a substantial amount of heat, the cooling fans tend to be noisy, and 30-s time lag is between turning the unit on and actual light emission[60]. These limitations can be centrally installed, with curing wands radiating into individual operatories. According to Powell *et al.*[39], the temperature increase within the pulp chamber has no significant pulpal risk when using the low limits of laser energy to cure composite resin. Chances of leaving the laser on the tooth long enough to damage the pulp are meager.

Cost: Cost of the argon laser curing unit is very high. On the basis of the manufacturer, portable argon curing lasers range from $12,000 to $20,000, and central installation may incur additional expenses. Added to the cost consideration is the fear of rapid obsolescence in an arena of rapid technological change.

Risk to surrounding tissues: When laser light hits a target, it may be absorbed, transmitted, scattered, or reflected. When it is transmitted, tissue boundaries are crossed and tissues other than the target material are irradiated. As a result, whenever a laser is used in the oral cavity, the dentist must determine the risk to surrounding tissues.

Temperature increase: In studies by Brenneise and Blankenau, *in vitro* using extracted human teeth and *in vitro* in dogs, a temperature rise was observed in the dentinal roof, the pulp chamber, and within the pulp itself when an argon laser was used to cure composite resin in cavity preparations[39,40]. When 10, 20, and 30 s exposure times were tested, minimal effect was observed after 10 and 20 s, whereas necrosis and disruption were noted 5 days after 30-s exposure[41].

Visual damage: The argon laser beam is in short wavelength blue light, which has the highest energy photons of any wavelength of visible light. Its energy level is only slightly less than that of ultraviolet light, which has a well-documented history of posing a biohazard. Consequently, extreme care must be exercised to avoid direct exposure of the patient's eyes, as it could result in immediate visual damage. In addition, indirect exposure by reflection could also harm the operator's eyes over time.

Advances

"Pulsed argon laser" may be a solution for the shrinkage problem. Pulsing or periodic interruption of the beam can be precisely control Light Emitting Diode in nanoseconds. The theory is that interruption of the beam allows the target material to cool between laser pulses, thus preventing overheating.

Argon lasers currently available in the market are the HGM dental 200, 300, and 400 series (HGM Medical Laser Systems, Salt Lake, UT). These are available only in 488-nm wavelengths for curing and tooth whitening purposes.

Curing Depths and Efficiency of Various Light Units: An Overview

In a study conducted by Strassler[4], two brands of three composite resin types were selected. The composite resins tested were the following:

1. Hybrid composite resin by Prisma TPH (Dentsply/Caulk) and Z-250 (3M)
2. Flowable composite resin by Revolution (Kerr) and Virtuoso Flowable (DenMat)
3. Microfill by Durafill (Hereaus-Kulzer) and Virtuoso Sculptable (DenMat)

Five specimens were prepared for each composite resin with each curing light. A sharp explorer penetration test was used to measure the depth of cure. Resistance to penetration was considered as cured. Penetration of the explorer tip was uncured. Using a digital micrometer (Mitutoyo Digimatic), we measured the depth of cure. The results were as follows:

1. The Rembrandt Sapphire Light (DenMat) yielded the deepest depth of cure combined with the shortest time for curing (3 s).
2. There was variation in the depth of cure dependent on light type and composite type.
3. The hybrid composite resins had the deepest depth of cures with all lights tested.
4. The depth of cure of different composite resins should be checked to determine the optimal cure with the light-curing unit.
5. Rembrandt Sapphire Plasma Arc Curing light cures several times faster compared to halogen and light-emitting diodes.

In a study, Sulaiman[42] showed the relationship of distance with the intensity of light associated with the curing depth in various light cure units. The inverse square law showed the decrease in light intensity four times of the increase in distance.

A systematic review by De Santis and Baldi[17] searched and identified 189 reports out of which 182 were excluded after reviewing the title and abstract and 2 articles were included after manual search. The study concluded that the light-emitting diodes offer equal or even better performance for curing nanocomposite resins as compared to quartz–tungsten–halogen light-curing units.

In another study conducted by Mills et al.[4], the higher curing depth was found for light-emitting diode light-curing unit than that for the halogen light-curing unit. This increase in depth of cure with the light-emitting diode was approximately 0.2 mm for each composite.

Caughman et al.[43] postulated clinical guidelines for photo-curing, showing secure polymerization of resin composites for layers <2 mm at 280 mW/cm². For quartz–tungsten–halogen light units and 3 mm layers, even at 800 mW/cm² and 80 s exposure time (energy density of 64,000 mW/cm²), no adequate polymerization was observed. These results raise question about the recommended bulk curing of plasma arc curable resin composites. A recent study has shown a linear relationship between light intensity of both quartz–tungsten–halogen and light-emitting diode lamps and curing depth. Interestingly, even prolonged curing times did not guarantee higher curing depths. Polymerization depth is affected if the light tip is placed at a distance of more than 6 mm from the resin composite surface[44]. At a distance of 12 mm from the light tip, no desirable curing of resin composites was accomplished, being independent of the type of light (quartz–tungsten–halogen vs. plasma arc curing) and the curing mode (soft start vs. standard)[45].

Effect of Curing Time and Curing Light Intensity on Light-Curing Units

Malhotra and Mala[1] showed the following factors could affect the clinical efficiency of various light-curing units:

- Factors related to resin-based composites
- Factors associated with light-curing units
- Factors associated with environment
- Other factors

Factors related to resin-based composites

1. *Type and concentration of fillers and other components*: The filler particles tend to scatter the light. Smaller particles have maximum scattering because the particle sizes correspond to the wavelength range of the photoinitiator. Therefore, the particle size should be controlled as it affects the color of composite.

2. *Shade of materials*: Darker shades or more opaque reins tend to absorb more light, thus requiring longer curing times.

3. *Type of photoinitiator*: Most composites contain CQ photoinitiators, which can cause an undesirable yellowing of the final aesthetics. Thus, whiter and more transparent compounds derived from acylphosphine oxides (e.g., MAPO) are being used.

Factors associated with light-curing units

1. *Size of the light-curing unit tip*: The decrease in unit tip size increases not only the light intensity but also the temperature. Thus, smaller tip units should be used with caution.

2. *Type of unit*: Light-emitting diode, quartz–tungsten–halogen, and so on.

3. *Exposure time*

4. *Light source*: Lamp output intensity should always be maintained for long use.

5. *Angulation of the tip*: A light beam produces a circular spot of light when held perpendicular to the restoration surface. With the change in angulation, the spot becomes elliptical and thus the intensity is reduced.

6. *Beam spreading*: The light beam disperses from its origin leading to an inhomogeneous distribution of light intensity. Thus, both the light intensity and amount of curing decreases as the tip is moved away.

7. *Color changes of composite*: A shade guide should be fabricated using cured resin samples as resin materials often show perceptible color changes during polymerization.

8. *Distance of curing tip from resin surface*

9. *Temperature rise during curing*

10. *Effect of autoclaving on light-curing unit tip*: During autoclaving, boiler scale tends to form on the instruments being sterilized, including the light-curing tip. This can compromise the intensity of irradiation transmitted from the source. This effect can be minimized by polishing the tip regularly between autoclaving processes.

11. *Degree of conversion/degree of cure*

Factors associated with environment

1. *Effect of surrounding atmosphere*: The air molecules scatter the light. Thus, the tip should be within 3 mm of the composite surface and within 1 mm for darker shades.

2. *Effect of ambient and operating light*: The operating light can initiate premature curing, thus reducing working time. The use of yellow filters and polyester-based photographic filters is effective in avoiding this unwanted activation and in extending the working time.

Other factors

Effect of tooth structure: The exposure time needs to be increased two- to fourfold when attempting to cure through tooth structure.

Curing time

For the incremental layering technique of resin composites, the maximum thickness of each individual composite layer recommended was <2 mm with a required curing time of 40 s for each layer. To achieve a maximum conversion rate, some authors recommended curing at lower intensities of 500 mW/cm² within extended polymerization intervals.

More recently, this paradigm was questioned constantly when facing high-output curing lights. Koran and Kurschner[46] evaluated the hardness, adhesion, shrinkage, viscosity, and degree of polymerization of the variables at different light intensities and different polymerization times with quartz–tungsten–halogen. At energy densities of 17,000 mW/cm², no further improvement of mechanical properties was feasible, leading to the conclusion that with latest generation light-emitting diode units providing output levels consistently between 1500 and 2000 mW/cm², polymerization time can be decreased to 20 s.

In the majority of surveys addressing curing light intensity and curing time in private dental offices, curing units often lack maintenance and thus provide weak performance, combined with curing times often being limited to 20 s. Therefore, compensation of these practically relevant problems by higher energy output may be the key point in recent photopolymerization technology.

On the basis of these observations and the surveys published, it was observed that most of the resin composite restorations in dental offices may not be sufficiently cured, with still having issues such as higher abrasion and less biocompatibility. This situation could be overcome in future with more durable and biocompatible resin composite restorations.

The following points outlined by Dr. Gordon Christensen, a world-renowned dental lecturer and educator, should be considered while curing:

1. Darker color resins require more curing time.
2. Thin-layer restorative resins or bonding agents require less curing time.
3. Microfills require more curing time than microhybrids, nanohybrids, or nanofills.
4. Ceramic requires more curing time.
5. The farther the light is from the resin being cured, the more the curing time.
6. Small flecks of cured resin or bonding agent attached to the curing tip decrease the light intensity, thus increasing the curing time. This debris should be removed with a sharp scalpel and then the end of the curing tip should be polished with composite polishing disks. Then, a 2-in.^{2} piece of household Saran wrap should be placed on the tip of the light. Replacing the wrap after each patient will help avoid accumulating another layer of debris on the tip.

Dr. Christensen also suggested that the shade and opacity of the composite should also be taken into consideration: "Darker and more opaque shades typically require longer curing times for a given thickness of composite. Recommended curing thicknesses are typically 2 mm, and it is reasonable to extend curing times by 50% for very dark shades, or reduce thickness by about 50%."

Curing intensity

Light activation with blue light is achieved at about 470 nm, which is usually absorbed by the photoinitiators such as CQ^3. The initiation system starts the polymerization process by forming free radical. When a free radical collides with a C=C in the resin monomer, it pairs with one of the electrons of the double bond converting the other member of the pair into a free radical, and thus the reaction continues. In light-cured systems, a light source of 468 nm ($\pm$20) excites CQ or another diketone into a triplet state that interacts with a nonaromatic tertiary amine, such as *N,N*-dimethylaminoethyl methacrylate. Ideally, this process continues until all the monomers are polymerized.). Dentists should know that high-intensity light-emitting diode curing lights may produce high temperatures that can damage pulp irreversibly. Given the various factors that affect the pulp during restorative treatments, an increase in temperature may cause irreversible damage.

On the basis of the methodology used, the study shows that the temperature increase in dentin was directly proportional to the light intensity of the light-emitting diode appliances. The high-intensity light-emitting diode appliances produced significantly higher temperature increases in dentin than the quartz–tungsten–halogen appliances, both during photopolymerization of resin composite and after 24 h.

L.E.D. Radiometer (Fig 6)

This device has the following functions:

- has a meter scale calibrated for light-emitting diode curing lights
- measures the intensity of the visible curing light from 0 to 2000 mW/cm^2
- measures only useful energy in the visible light spectrum range between 400 and 500 nm
- requires no battery powered by curing light source

- accommodates light guides with the tip diameters from 7 to 13 mm

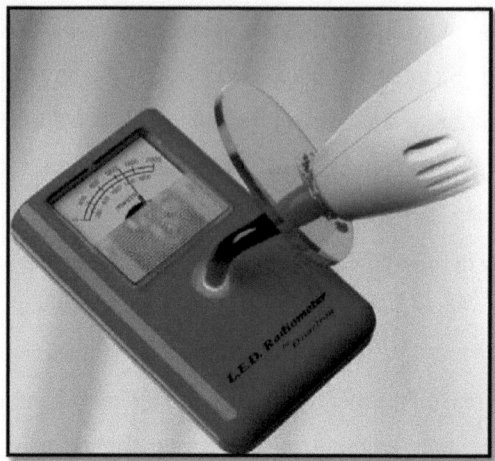

Fig. 6. L.E.D. Radiometer

Temperature Rise Induced by Light-Curing Units

Soares *et al.*[50] reported that the main irradiation produced by light-curing lamps is in the infrared spectrum region, which is absorbed by the composite, resulting in greater molecular vibration and heat generation. Heat-absorbing filters decrease the passage of infrared energy to the tooth when the light passes through them. The light-emitting diode was developed to reduce the heat emission. In an *in vivo* experiment by Zach and Cohen[68], when teeth of Rhesus monkey were subjected to temperature changes, irreversible pulpitis was observed inside the pulp chamber. In a study by Dogan *et al.*[26], rise in temperature induced by various light-curing units through human dentin was measured. Light-emitting diode light-curing units produced the lowest rise in temperature. Examining different modes of light-emitting diode, it was found that the soft-start mode produced the highest rise in temperature and that the temperature values produced by this polymerization technique were significantly higher than those by the standard mode in all the specimens with the same dentin thickness ($p <$ 0.05).

In an article published in *Dental Economics*, Dr. Christensen suggested a simple heat test for dentists and dental staff who are shifting to faster curing. He recommended placing the tip of the light guide of the curing light on the small fingernail, turning the light on, and holding the light on the fingernail until the heat can no longer be tolerated. The heat soon builds up and in about 3 s, the light has to be removed from the fingernail because of the discomfort. After accomplishing that simple test, he suggested applying the same logic when curing resin in teeth.

Bagis *et al.*[49] measured temperature changes from the heat generated by three commercially available light-curing units. The study evaluated the heat generation of three types of light-curing units including the following:

1. Quartz-tungsten-halogen curing light at 500 mW/cm² (Hilux Smartlite; Benlioglu Dental, Turkey).

2. Plasma arc curing unit at over 1800 mW/cm² (Plasma Star SP-2000; Monitex, Taiwan).

3. Light-emitting diode curing unit at 600 mW/cm² (LedMax 550; Benlioglu Dental).

For every test period, the highest rises in temperature (54.4 ± 1.65°C) occurred during activation of a plasma arc curing unit. The least temperature increase (11.8 ± 1.3°C) occurred with a light-emitting diode for each tested period, except for the measurement of the temperature rise using the quartz-tungsten-halogen curing unit at 10-s interval. The results show that the choice of light activation unit and curing time is important when polymerizing light-activated, resin-based restorations to avoid any thermal damage to the pulp.

Zach and Cohen[47] stated that a temperature rise of 5.5°C within the pulp chamber would lead to irreversible pulp damage. Thus, the earlier-mentioned findings must be taken into consideration while using and choosing the light-curing unit.

Selection and Maintenance of Light-Curing Units

Selection

No single best visible light–curing unit is available because different units work differently for different applications. Performance of the unit depends on the type of material used and its curing guidelines recommended by the manufacturer. A unit with a larger diameter of cure saves chair time by curing larger portions of composites and veneers during each curing cycle. Several factors that must be considered before purchasing a visible light–curing unit are as follows:

1. Maximum diameter of curing tip
2. Heat generation by curing unit
3. Ease of use of controls and timer
4. Durability of curing tips to sterilization
5. Size and portability of unit
6. Voltage regulation
7. Price and performance ratio

Performance surveys published worldwide on light-curing units used in dental offices have shown that many deliver intensity less than 300 mW/cm², which is unsatisfactory for light curing and is likely due to inadequate maintenance. In addition, the light tips of many light-curing units were either damaged or covered in resin, which also contribute to the reduction in light output. Clinicians should regularly check their light-curing units for adequate output and inspect the light tip for any damage or debris before each use.

Spectral emission

For a quartz–tungsten–halogen light-curing unit, the range of wavelengths is sufficiently broad to adequately polymerize any resin-based dental composites. However, most light-emitting diode units produce a very narrow spectral emission[70] and are usually optimized to cure the commonly used CQ photoinitiator that is most reactive to light at ~468 nm. Some resin-based composites use alternative photoinitiators that require very different wavelengths (~410 nm), thus it is possible to use a light-emitting diode unit that is not ideally matched to the resin-based composites. Recently, broadband light-emitting diode units have been introduced that use two or more colors of light-emitting diodes, which suggests that their spectral output includes both blue (~460 nm) and violet (~410 nm) wavelengths of light. These lights can polymerize resin-based composites containing both conventional and alternative photoinitiators. However, in some polywave light-emitting diode units, the spectral emission distribution is not uniform across the light tip. Thus, some areas of the resin may not receive the required wavelengths.

Irradiance value

Irradiance from a light-curing unit, also referred to as power density, is usually expressed in mW/cm^2. However, the light output from dental light-curing units is not uniformly distributed over the end of the light tip. Conventional methods of measuring the light output (such as a dental radiometer, a thermopile, or an integrating sphere) do not the extent of uniformness of the light beam, and, in fact, may be misleading because a single irradiance value does not show if "hot spots" are present within the light beam. This problem is more with light-emitting diode units than with quartz–tungsten–halogen units. Manufacturers should provide the beam profile from their light-curing unit over clinically relevant distances (0–8 mm), as provided by some now[50].

Irradiance over distance

In some light-curing units, the irradiance may be high near the tip, but then it drastically decreases with the increase in distance from the tip. Clinicians need to analyze data that report the output or performance of the light-curing units not only at 0 mm from the tip but also at clinically relevant distances. Manufacturers and researchers have now started providing this information.

Maintenance

Several features need be taken into consideration ensuring a visible light–curing unit to operate at full capacity[51]:

1. *Curing tip*: Accumulation of composite at the curing tip can reduce light intensity to a great extent. It occurs when the curing tip comes into contact with the composite during curing. The ideal curing distance is 1 mm. Demetron offers a cleaning kit to eliminate this buildup.

2. *Fiber-optic cords*: The fibers of fiber-optic bundles are brittle that break on repetitive bending. Procedures and storage that unnecessarily bend the cords should be avoided.

3. *Light guides*: The tips of light guides should be shiny and free of materials. For most light guides, autoclaving can be used, but it may eventually cause some degradation, which is observed as cloudiness at the ends of the fibers. "Boiler scale" results from repeated autoclaving of rigid light guides.

4. *Filters*: A filter is present in most of the curing units that selects the appropriate wavelength to block glare, heat, light, and any unused energy during the curing process. This filter is usually located between the curing bulb and the cord tip or gun rod. The filters must be checked regularly for any pit, crack, or peel, and should be replaced as needed.

5. *Fans*: The fan should be kept clean by vacuuming the exhaust port where it is mounted. For this purpose, there is no need to take the curing unit apart. The smaller fans used in many gun-type units may need periodic replacement because of wear on the bearings. Worn bearings are noisy; noise is a warning of potential fan failure. The manufacturer should immediately replace a noisy fan. A unit should not be operated if its fan stops functioning.

Problems Associated with Light-Curing Units

There are several problems related to the light-curing units. Some of these have been summarized as follows:

1. *Bulb frosting*: According to Antonson and Benedetto[52], bulbs become frosted when the glass enclosing the filament becomes cloudy or white. This is due to deposition of metal oxides, which vaporize and form a film on the glass bulb. Frosting can decrease the output of curing light by 45%.

2. *Reflector degradation*: According to Ham *et al.*[53], reflector degradation is a result of the reflector film loss or development of a white or yellow coating of oxides on the reflector surface. This can decrease the output of curing light by 66%, gradually leading to complete loss of intensity. In general, light-emitting diodes have fewer problems related to maintenance than halogen bulbs but must be checked for decreased power density due to heat accumulation during long curing times. Heat can also lead to degeneration of light-emitting diode over time.

3. *Radiometers*: It is a specialized light meter that quantifies blue light output. It determines the effectiveness of a curing unit by measuring the intensity of 468-nm light coming out of the light guide tip. These are sold as small handheld devices or may be built into curing units. To obtain a baseline for future reference, it is important to test a curing light when it is new. Most

radiometers measure the intensity of light in the 400–500 mm bandwidth, which is broader than is required by most photoinitiators and makes these units less reliable in evaluating curing units with narrower spectral outputs (i.e., light-emitting diodes and lasers). A precise measurement of any unit's spectral bandwidth is expected from a specialized radiometer capable of measuring a narrower bandwidth of around 468 nm.

4. *Ocular hazards of curing lights*: The blue light used to polymerize composite is not well tolerated by the human eye. All light-cured polymerization systems use light that is harmful to vision[1]. Many studies by Ham et al.[53] and Chamorro et al.[54] showed that blue light can damage the retina. Blue light has been found to form free radicals in the eye, in a similar manner as it does in composite resins. However, in the retina, these free radicals react with the water content of cells, leading to the formation of peroxides. These peroxides are reactive and denature the delicate photoreceptors of the eye.

5. *Solar retinitis*: Satrom et al.[55] estimated that blue light is 33 times more damaging to the photoreceptors of the retina than is the ultraviolet light. The severity of burns increases with the increase in exposure duration. This damage is known as "solar retinitis." Some laboratory studies indicate that exposure of less than 2 min to visible light–curing units (total daily dose from 25 cm) may be safe[56]. Younger eyes are more susceptible to blue light damage. It is important to educate staff about this so they can ensure that children are prevented from staring at curing lamps during treatment. The resulting damage could be profound and lifelong.

Eye Protection

Albers[51] has provided the following instructions for eye safety:
- To avoid looking at the curing light source completely.

- To cover the curing site with a dark object.

- To cover the curing site with the hand; this may prove to be an unsafe practice.

- To cover the curing field with the reflective side of a mouth mirror. This prevents excess blue light from reflecting back against the restorative and improves curing.

If looking at the light source for placement is unavoidable, then eye protection is warranted. Unfortunately, most optical glasses and plastic contact lenses transmit blue light and near-ultraviolet light radiation with little attenuation. Many colored plastic glasses and handheld shields are available (Fig. 7). The effectiveness of a light shield can be tested easily. The wavelengths that harm the eye are the same ones that cure composite. To test a shield (or pair of protective glasses), try to cure the composite by shining the curing light through the shield onto the composite.

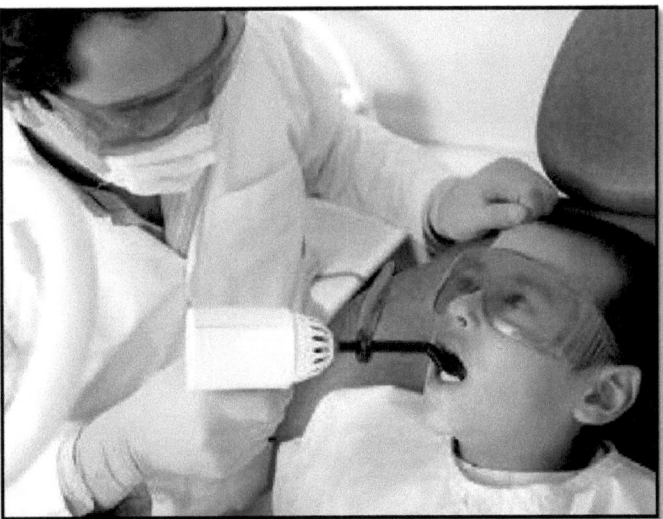

Fig. 7. Curing-light protective glasses

Retinal burning and advancement of macular degeneration are potential risks while using light-curing units. Therefore, clinicians should use protective reddish-orange eyewear or shields that act as "blue blockers" to help prevent potential problems. Extended exposure (100 s) of the macaque retina to blue light (400–500 nm) produces a photochemical type or types of lesion. The basic mechanisms responsible for such photic damage are not known, but the toxic combination of light and oxygen leading to the formation of free radicals ($O_2^{\cdot-}$, H_2O_2, $OH\cdot$, and $O^{\cdot}$) has been suggested as a possible source of the phototoxicity.

In normal vision, visual pigments absorb light to split or convert the pigment and bleach the photoreceptor cells of the retina. In the case of blue light, this process is considered to be mediated by rhodopsin, the visual pigment present in the rods. Phototransduction (the process by which light is converted into electrical signals) is triggered by the conversion of *cis* retinal to the intermediate all-*trans* retinal in rhodopsin. On a cellular level, rhodopsin activation by blue light can induce oxidant injury in both the inner and the outer segments of the rods. The degree of damage is proportional to the amount of light absorbed. When the photoreceptor cell is bleached, it is unavailable for light absorption until the visual pigment is reformed through a metabolic process called the visual cycle[57].

Blue light can, however, bypass the visual cycle and restore rhodopsin from its bleached state through a process called photoreversal. This enables rhodopsin molecules to absorb even more blue light, thus greatly increasing the potential for retinal damage. An important determinant for rhodopsin regeneration is the retinal pigment epithelium protein 65 because blue light has been found to have no effect on retinas when rhodopsin regeneration is inhibited by the depletion of retinal pigment epithelium protein 65 in mice[58].

Three light-sensitive pigments are present in retinal cones, which are maximally sensitive to short (blue), medium (green), or long (red) wavelengths. Colors are detected when the three photopigments are stimulated to different degrees; white and gray can be recognized on equal stimulation of all three photopigments. Deficiencies in color perception can be congenital or acquired, and the latter can be attributed to ocular pathology, intracranial injury, or prolonged use of therapeutic drugs. Repeated exposure to blue argon light can slowly cause small losses of color contrast sensitivity in ophthalmologists, with a correlation between the number of years of laser experience and a chronic reduction in tritan color contrast sensitivity[59]

Composites represent one of the many modern restorative materials in dentistry. Their biggest advantage is that they are lightweight yet strong. By choosing appropriate combination of matrix and filler, we can make a new material that exactly meets the requirements of a particular application.

Curing of composites is a complex mechanism. The light is used to activate the photoinitiator system in light-curing unit. The detailed light-emitting diode description of the curing mechanism has been discussed in detail. Techniques such as "soft-start polymerization" have been used recently to reduce the polymerization shrinkage. The light-curing units have been classified according to their generations, gun-type units and countertop units.

Different light-curing protocols are available such as soft start, step curing, or oscillating irradiation. These special curing modes have been taken into consideration to increase the degree of conversion for better material properties and to reduce internal stress for better marginal quality in bonded resin composite restorations. Light-curing dental materials undergo polymerization by photoinitiators. Camphorquinone is one of the major photoinitiators of composite resin, which reacts most efficiently between 410 and 490 nm.

The first photocuring units were designed to emit ultraviolet light (about 365 nm) through a quartz rod from a high-pressure mercury source. These units were introduced in the early 1970s. The problems associated with the use of ultraviolet light include the retinal damage and inability of these units to cure deep into the restorations.

Dr. Mohammed Bassoiuny (Turner School of Dentistry, Manchester) placed the first visible light–cured composite restoration on Dr. John Yearn, the then head of department. The team of engineers at General Electric developed the quartz–tungsten–halogen light source for use in aircraft lights, where small but very bright and durable sources were needed. The advantages of using visible light were that 2-mm-thick increments could typically be placed using 40–60 s exposure from a quartz–tungsten–halogen light source, and that the potential formation of cataracts and oral microflora alteration were minimized. However, direct retinal burning and advancement of macular degeneration were now a potential for ocular damage, as the wavelength necessary for initiating the visible light–initiated systems was directly within the frequencies known to cause immediate and permanent damage resulting from retinal burning.

The plasma arc curing units were developed in the mid-1960s. Initially, these units were not used for dental purposes but to provide broad-banded radiation for visualization of operating fields (e.g., endoscopy and colonoscopy) as well as for minimally invasive medical procedures. The only advantage of these units is the shorter polymerization time; however, they have low efficacy and high-temperature development.

The problems associated with all earlier used light-curing units led to the introduction of light-emitting diodes into restorative dentistry. Light-emitting diode technology has advanced significantly since blue light–emitting diodes were adopted for curing composites. Newer light-emitting diodes (such as L.E. Demetron and Coltolux light-emitting diode) use a high-intensity blue light–emitting diode containing a large semiconductor crystal, which increases both the illuminated area and the light intensity. The higher light intensity and narrow spectrum make these devices more efficient than the conventional quartz–tungsten–halogen units. "G-light" by GC is one of the recent developments in the field of light-emitting diodes for the curing of restorative materials. The light emits two wavelength radiations that cure faster and more efficiently. According to Zach and Cohen[47], light-emitting diodes convert electrical power into visible blue light efficiently, without generating the large amount of heat associated with halogen lamps. Thus, these are preferred over the other light sources.

In 1960, Theodore H. Maiman developed the first laser—a pulsed ruby laser. The argon-ion laser was marketed first to enhance the effects of vital tooth bleaching in Europe, and it is still used for that purpose. The thoroughness and depth of composite resin polymerization are greater with laser than with visible light–curing units. Argon laser–cured resins have less unpolymerized monomer compared to those cured with visible light–curing units. Kameyama et al.[37] showed that gallium nitride–based violet laser diode (VLM500) can also be used for curing purposes. The research for new lasers is still on.

The temperature inside the pulp chamber rises due to activation of composites by light sources, which might cause pulpal damage. Various in vitro studies have shown that the thermal variations occurring during light curing could depend on the photoactivation methods/dentin thickness[60]. Studies have shown that in pulp tissue a temperature rise of 5–6°C caused necrosis in 15% cases, 11.2°C in 60% cases, and 11.8°C in 100% cases. According to the study conducted by Dogan et al.[48], high-power light-emitting diodes could be used to attain temperature rises lower than the critical value, which cause pulpal injury. Among the three modes of light-emitting diode used, the soft-start mode registered the highest temperature rise ($p < 0.05$) in all the test conditions. The difference in total energy produced by these three modes could have also accounted for the different changes in temperature. The soft-start mode produced total energy of 22 J/cm^2, whereas the other two modes produced 11 J/cm^2. On the basis of these results, it could be said that the standard and/or pulse modes of light-emitting diode might reduce the risk of pulpal injury even in the case of thin dentin tissue. This was because these modes of light-emitting diode produced a lower temperature rise not only when compared with the soft-start mode but also against the standard curing mode of quartz–tungsten–halogen and plasma arc curing light-curing units used in this study.

Table 1 lists the advantages and disadvantages of various light-curing units.

Light-Curing Units	Advantages	Disadvantages
HALOGEN	Low-cost technology	Low efficiency
	Longest history in dental industry	Short service life
		High temperatures (lamp must be cooled by ventilating fan)
		Continuous spectrum must be narrowed by filter systems
PAC	Short polymerization times (no unambiguous scientific data to confirm this)	Very low efficiency

		High-temperature development (lamp is situated in the base unit and cooled by a ventilating fan)
		Continuous spectrum must be narrowed by filter systems
		High price
LASER	Low heat generation	Negative perception about curing quality due to high curing speeds
		Incompatible with some adhesives and composites
		Large base needed for power suppliers and cooling
		High price
LED	No need for filter systems	Due to their narrow emission spectrum, LEDs can only polymerize materials with an

	absorption maximum between 440 and 480 and camphorquinone as the photoinitiator
High efficiency leads to minimal heat (no ventilation fan required) and low power consumption (battery operation is possible)	Relatively new technology in the dental industry
Frame can be easily cleaned, because no slots for ventilation fan are needed	
Long service life	
Consistent output, with no bulbs to change	
Quiet	

PAC, plasma arc curing unit; LED, light-emitting diode.

Table 1. Advantages and disadvantages of various light-curing units

The introduction of step curing may be interpreted as the first attempt to reduce initial shrinking stress by delaying the gel phase[61,62]. During the pregel phase, the resin composite flows, and the stresses within the structures are relieved[63]. After gelation, flow ceases and cannot compensate for shrinkage stresses. Using step curing, the polymerization process is started for 10 s with low-level intensity ($100 \ mW/cm^2$). Consecutively, the light unit automatically increases the power output to 700 mW/cm^2. First results were promising and indicated less polymerization stress compared to conventional quartz–tungsten–halogen curing; however, after 10 years, no unanimous proof for improved marginal adaptation could be found[64]. Soft-start polymerization means also starting at a lower level (100 mW/cm^2); however, the increase to the final power density (800 mW/cm^2) takes an exponential curve. This special curing protocol is offered with different quartz–tungsten–halogen and light-emitting diode models. Nevertheless, the effectiveness of soft-start curing is not unanimously clarified. However, a certain reduction of polymerization stresses was shown[65,66]. Only in Class V cavities, some positive effects were reported[67]. The pulse-activated polymerization uses high-intensity short impulses (e.g., eLight: 10 pulses for 2 s each 750 mW/cm^2). To date, no enhanced polymerization kinetics has been found. The so-called pulse-delay technique was repeatedly investigated *in vitro*. With this technique, the restoration is initially irradiated with short pulses of light energy (pre-polymerization at low light, e.g., 3 or 20 s with 100 mW/cm^2).

Apart from the type of the light-curing unit used, the clinician's knowledge and skill in handling these materials contributes to polymerization and final result of the resin-based composite. According to Malhotra and Mala[1], the clinical tips that may help in proper curing are as follows:

1. Composition and shade should be considered while selecting a light-curing unit.
2. The light-curing unit should be stepped across a large restoration.
3. A 2-mm increment should be cured considering appropriate *R* value.
4. Yellow or polyester-based photographic filters should be used to extend the working time.

5. Exposure time is to be increased two or three times when curing through tooth structure. Light-transmitting wedges and focusing tips should be used.

6. The mirror should be routinely cleaned and the unit tips should be polished to preserve the reflection effectiveness of the light-curing unit. Output intensity, energy density, and beam spreading of the light-curing unit should be checked.

Appropriately polymerized material will have a positive influence on both the physical and biological properties of the restoration and should aid in promoting clinical success. This book has focused on various light-curing units available today. The never-ending advancements in the field of conservative dentistry encouraged us to investigate and document about this topic. Advancements in the light-curing units have continuously followed the advances in the restorative materials.

1.   Malhotra N, Mala K. Light-curing considerations for resin-based composite materials: A review. Part I. Compendium of Continuing Education in Dentistry 2010;31(7):498–505.

2.   Pilo R, Oelgiesser D, Cardash HS. A survey of output intensity and potential for depth of cure among light-curing units in clinical use. Journal of Dentistry 1999;27:235–241.

3.   Safarcherati H, Alaghehmand H. Hardness of composite resin polymerized with different light-curing units. Caspian Journal of Dental Research 2012;1(1):32–35.

4.   Strassler HE. Cure depths using different light units. *DentalTown Magazine* August 2002:22–24.

5.   Mills RW, Jandt KD, Ashworth SH. Dental composite depth of cure with halogen and blue light emitting diode technology. British Dental Journal 1999;186(8):388–391.

6.   Leonard DL, Charlton DG, Roberts HW, Cohen ME. Polymerization efficiency of Light Emitting Diode curing lights. Journal of Esthetic and Restorative Dentistry 2002;14(5):286–295.

7.   Neumann M, Schmitt CC, Ferreira GC, Corrêa IC. The initiating radical yields and the efficiency of polymerization for various dental photoinitiators excited by different light curing units. Dental Materials 2006;22(6):576–584.

8.   Apicella A, Apicella D, Sorrentino R, Ferro F, Perillo L, Gherlone E. Effect of plasma and halogen light-curing units on shrinkage stress phenomena. International Dentistry 2008;10(3):42–48.

9.   Singh TK, Ataide I, Fernandes M, Lambor RT. Light curing devices—a
        clinical review. Journal of Orofacial Research 2011;1(1):15–19.

10.   Rueggeberg FA. State of the art: dental photocuring—a review. Dental
        Materials 2011;27:39–52.

11.   Hunt PR. Microconservative restorations for approximal carious lesions.
        Journal of American Dental Association 1990;120(1):37–40.

12.   Park J, Chang J, Ferracane J, Lee IB. How should composite be layered to
        reduce shrinkage stress: incremental or bulk filling? Dental Materials
        2008;24:1501–1505.

13.   Lutz F, Krejci I, Oldenburg TR. Elimination of polymerization stresses at
        the margins of posterior composite resin restorations: a new restorative
        technique. Quintessence International 1986;17(2):777–784.

14.   Ciucchi B, Bouillaguet S, Jacques H. Proximal adaptation and marginal
        seal of posterior composite resin restorations placed with direct and
        indirect techniques. Quintessence International 1990;21(8):663–669.

15.   Davidson CL, De Gee AJ. Relaxation of polymerization contraction
        stresses by flow in dental composites. Journal of Dental Research
        1984;63(2):146–148.

16.   Sandner B, Kammer S, Wartewig S. Crosslinking copolymerization of
        epoxy methacrylates as studied by Fourier transform Raman spectroscopy.
        Polymer 1996;37(21):4705–4712.

17.   De Santis A, Baldi M. Photo-polymerisation of composite resins measured
        by micro-Raman spectroscopy. Polymer 2004;45(11):3797–3804.

18.   Silikas N, Eliades G, Watts DC. Light intensity effects on resin-composite degree of conversion and shrinkage strain. Dental Materials 2000;16(4):292–296.

19.   Soares LES, Rocha R, Martin AA, Pinheiro LB, Zampieri M. Monomer conversion of composite dental resins photoactivated by a halogen lamp and a LED: an FT-Raman spectroscopy study. Quimica Nova 2005;28(2):229–232.

20.   Soares LES, Martin AA, Pinheiro ALB. Degree of conversion of composite resin: A Raman study. Journal of Clinical Laser Medicine and Surgery 2005;21(6):357–362.

21.   Yoon TH, Lee YK, Lim BS, Kim CW. Degree of polymerization of resin composites by different light sources. Journal of Oral Rehabilitation 2002;29(12):1165–1173.

22.   Tarle Z, Meniga A, Knezević A, Sutalo J, Ristić M, Pichler G. Composite conversion and temperature rise using a conventional, plasma arc, and an experimental blue LED curing unit. Journal of Oral Rehabilitation 2002;29(7):662–667.

23.   Knezevic A, Tarle Z, Meniga A, Sutalo J, Pichler G, Ristić M. Degree of conversion and temperature rise during polymerization of composite resin samples with blue diodes. Journal of Oral Rehabilitation 2001;28(6):586–591.

24.   Soares LES, Rocha R, Martin AA, Pinheiro LB, Zampieri M. Monomer conversion of composite dental resins photoactivated by a halogen lamp and a LED: an FT-Raman spectroscopy study. Quimica Nova 2005;28(2):229–232.

25. Miyazaki M, Hattori T, Ichiishi Y, Kondo M, Onose H, Moore BK.. Evaluation of curing units used in private dental offices. Operative dentistry. 1998;23(2):50–54.

26. Kramer N, Lohbauer U, García-Godoy F, Frankenberger R. Light curing of resin-based composites in the LED era. American Journal of Dentistry. 2008;21(3):135–142.

27. Pettemerides AP, Sherriff M, Ireland AJ. An In Vivo study to compare a plasma arc light and a conventional quartz halogen curing light in orthodontic bonding. European Journal of Orthodontics 2004;26(6):573–577.

28. Brackett WW, Haisch LD, Covey DA. Effect of plasma arc curing units on the microleakage of class V resin-based composite restoration. American Journal of Dentistry 2000;13:121–122.

29. Oyama N, Komori A, Nakahara R. Evaluation of Light Curing Units Used for Polymerization of Orthodontic Bonding Agents. Angle Orthodontist 2004;74(6):810–815.

30. The Dental Advisor. LE Oyama N, Komori A, Nakahara R. Evaluation of Light Curing Units Used for Polymerization of Orthodontic Bonding Agents. Angle Orthodontist 2004;74(6):810–815.

31. D light-curing units. Journal of the Canadian Dental Association 2005;71(10):710–711.

32. The latest in LED technology. British Dental Journal 2010;209:146–114.

33. Corciolani G, Vichi A, Swift EJ. Turbo tips. Journal of Esthetic and Restorative Dentistry 2011;23(5):294–295.

34.   Harris DM, Pick RM. Laser Physics Chicago. Journal of Canadian Dental
       Association 1999; 65:447-450.

35.   Blankenau RJ, Kelsey WP, Powell GL, Shearer GO, Barkmeier WW,
       Cavel WT. Degree of composite resin polymerization with visible light and
       argon laser. American Journal of Dentistry 1991;4(1):40–42.

36.   Dederich DN. Laser/tissue interaction: what happens to laser light when it
       strikes tissue? Journal of the American Dental Association 1993;124:57–
       61.

37.   Kameyama A, Hatayama H, Kato J, Haruyama A, Teraoka H, Takase Y,
       et al. Light-curing of dental resins with GaN violet laser diode: the effect
       of photoinitiator on mechanical strength. Lasers in Medical Science
       2011;26(3):279–283.

38.   Intraoral resin curing lights. Clinical Research Associates Newsletter
       1996;20:1–2.

39.   Powell GL, Morton TH, Whisenant BK. Argon laser oral safety parameters
       for teeth. Lasers in Surgery and Medicine 1993;13(5):548–552.

40.   Anic I, Pavelic B, Peric B, Matsumoto K. In vitro pulp chamber
       temperature rises associated with argon laser polymerization of composite
       resin. Lasers in Surgery and Medicine 1996;19(4):438–444.

41.   Brenneise CV, Blankenau RJ. Response of associated oral soft tissues
       when exposed to argon laser during polymerization of dental resins. Lasers
       in Surgery and Medicine 1997;20(4):467–472.

42.   Sulaiman JMA. Analysis of intensity in different light cure units used in
       dentistry. Al-Rafidain Dental Journal 2010;10(1):192–197.

43. Caughman WF, Rueggeberg FA, Curtis JW. Clinical guidelines for photocuring restorative resins. Journal of the American Dental Association 1995;126:1280–1282.

44. Lindberg A, Peutzfeldt A, Van Dijken JW. Curing depths of a universal hybrid and a flowable resin composite cured with quartz tungsten halogen and light-emitting diode units. Acta Odontologica Scandinavica 2004;62(2):97–101.

45. Caldas DB, de Almeida JB, Correr-Sobrinho L, Sinhoreti MA, Consani S. Influence of curing tip distance on resin composite Knoop hardness number, using three different light curing units. Operative Dentistry 2003;28(3):315–320.

46. Koran P, Kurschner R. Effects of sequential versus continuous irradiation of a light-cured resin composite on shrinkage, viscosity, adhesion, and degree of polymerization. American Journal of Dentistry 1998;11(1):17–22.

47. Zach L, Cohen G. Pulp response to externally applied heat. Oral Surgery, Oral Medicine, and Oral Pathology 1965:19:515–530.

48. Dogan A, Hubbezoglu I, Dogan OM, Bolayir G, Demir H. Temperature rise induced by various light curing units through human dentin. Dental Materials Journal 2009;28(3):253–260.

49. Bagis B, Bagis Y, Ertas E, Ustaomer S. Comparison of the heat generation of light curing units. Journal of Contemporary Dental Practice 2008;9(2):1–9.

50. 3M ESPE. *Paradigm™ LED Curing Light: Technical Data Sheet*. 3M ESPE Dental Products, St. Paul, MN; 2011.

51.   Albers HF. *Tooth-Colored Restoratives: Principles and Techniques.* Hamilton, ON: BC Decker; 2002:103–104.

52.   Antonson DE, Benedetto MD. Longitudinal intensity variability of visible light curing units. Quintessence International 1986;17(12):819–823.

53.   Ham WT, Mueller HA, Ruffolo JJ Jr, Millen JE, Cleary SF, Guerry RK, et al. Basic mechanisms underlying the production of photochemical lesions in the mammalian retina. Current Eye Research 1984;3(1):165–174.

54.   Chamorro E, Bonnin-Arias C, Pérez-Carrasco MJ, Muñoz de Luna J, Vázquez D, Sánchez-Ramos C. Effects of light-emitting diode radiations on human retinal pigment epithelial cells in vitro. American Society of Photobiology 2013;89(2):468–473.

55.   Satrom KD, Morris MA, Crigger LP. Potential retinal hazards of visible-light photo-polymerization units. Journal of Dental Research 1987;66(3):731–736.

56.   Griess GA, Blankenstein MF. Additivity and repair of actinic retinal lesions. Investigative Ophthalmology & Visual Science 1981;20(6):803–807.

57.   Algvere PV, Marshall J, Seregard S. Age-related maculopathy and the impact of blue light hazard. Acta Ophthalmologica Scandinavica 2006;84(1):4–15.

58.   Demontis GC, Longoni B, Marchiafava PL. Molecular steps involved in light-induced oxidative damage to retinal rods. Investigative Ophthalmology & Visual Science 2002;43(7):2421–2427.

59.   Berninger TA, Canning CR, Gündüz K, Strong N, Arden GB. Using argon laser blue light reduces ophthalmologists' color contrast sensitivity. Argon

blue and surgeon's vision. Archives of Ophthalmology 1989;107:1453–1458.

60. Price RB, Labrie D, Whalen JM, Felix CM. Effect of distance on irradiance and beam homogeneity from 4 light-emitting diode curing units. Journal of the Canadian Dental Association 2011;77:9–11.

61. Ernst CP, Kurschner R, Willershausen B. Stress reduction in composite resin by means of a two-step polymerization unit. A photoelastic investigation. Acta Medica Denta Helvetica 1997;2:208–215.

62. Yap AU, Ng SC, Siow KS. Soft-start polymerization: influence on effectiveness of cure and post-gel shrinkage. Operative Dentistry 2001;26(3):260–266.

63. Feilzer AJ, De Gee AJ, Davidson CL. Setting stress in composite resin in relation to configuration of the restoration. Journal of Dental Research. 1987;66(11):1636–1639.

64. Muangmingsuk A, Senawongse P, Yudhasaraprasithi S. Influence of different soft-start polymerization techniques on marginal adaptation of Class V restorations. American Journal of Dentistry 2003;16(2):117–119.

65. Hofmann N, Hugo B, Klaiber B. Effect of irradiation type (LED or QTH) on photo-activated composite shrinkage strain kinetics, temperature rise, and hardness. European Journal of Oral Sciences 2002;110(6):471–479.

66. Soh MS, Yap AU, Siow KS. Post-gel shrinkage with different modes of LED and halogen light curing units. Operative Dentistry 2004;29(3):317–324.

67.   Mehl A, Hickel R, Kunzelmann KH. Physical properties and gap formation of light-cured composites with and without 'softstart-polymerization'. Journal of Dentistry 1997;25(3-4):321–330.

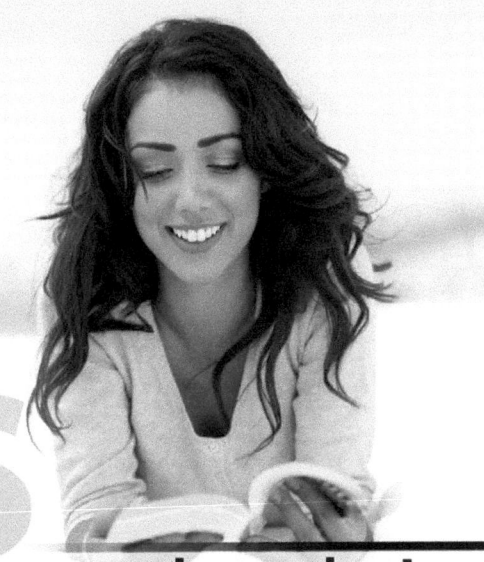

i **want** morebooks!

Buy your books fast and straightforward online - at one of the world's fastest growing online book stores! Environmentally sound due to Print-on-Demand technologies.

Buy your books online at
www.get-morebooks.com

Kaufen Sie Ihre Bücher schnell und unkompliziert online – auf einer der am schnellsten wachsenden Buchhandelsplattformen weltweit!
Dank Print-On-Demand umwelt- und ressourcenschonend produziert.

Bücher schneller online kaufen
www.morebooks.de

OmniScriptum Marketing DEU GmbH
Heinrich-Böcking-Str. 6-8
D - 66121 Saarbrücken
Telefax: +49 681 93 81 567-9

info@omniscriptum.de
www.omniscriptum.de

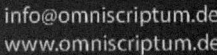
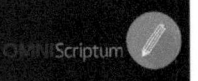

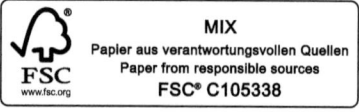

MIX
Papier aus verantwortungsvollen Quellen
Paper from responsible sources
FSC® C105338

Printed by Books on Demand GmbH, Norderstedt / Germany